What Really Happened to the Hat and the Gloves

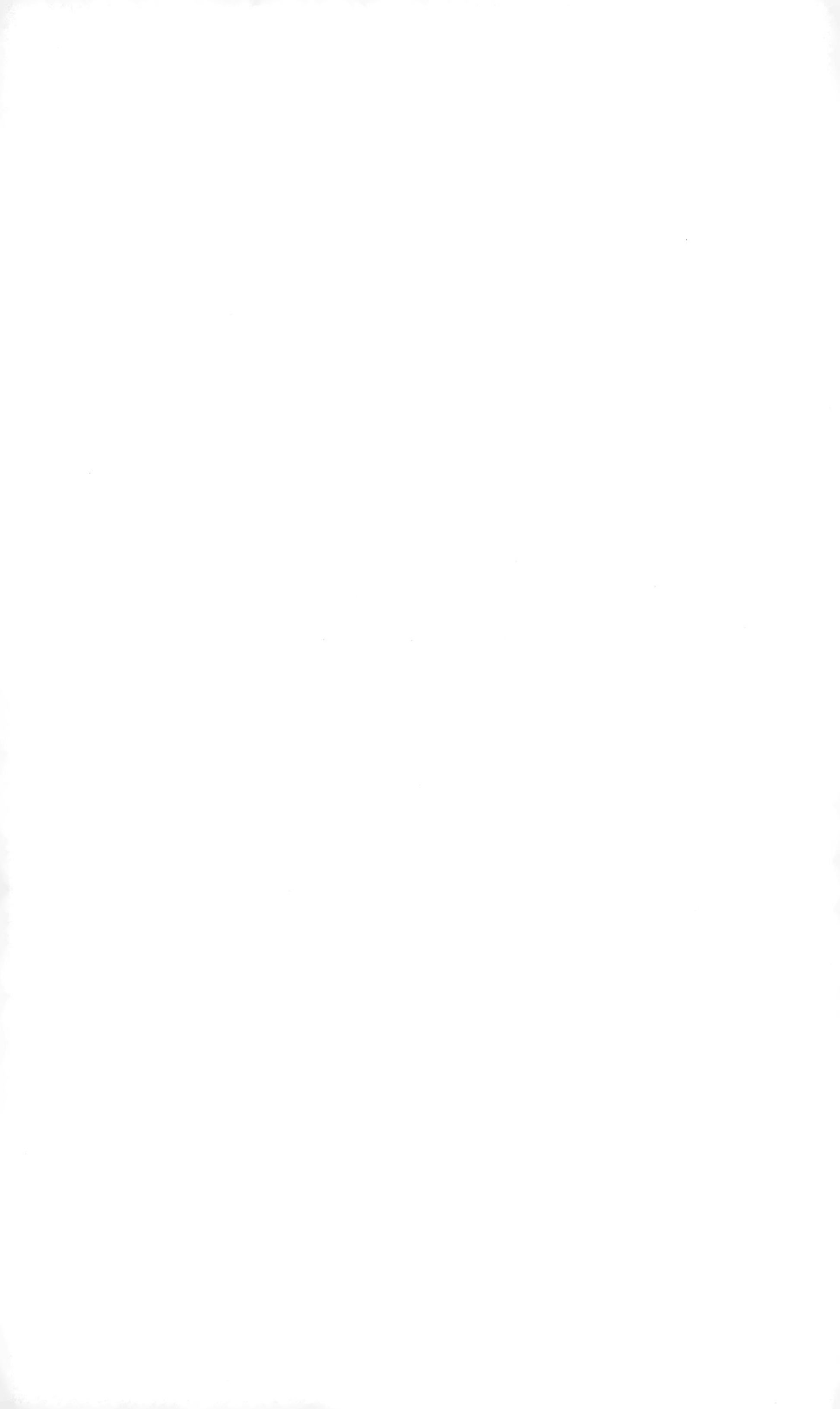

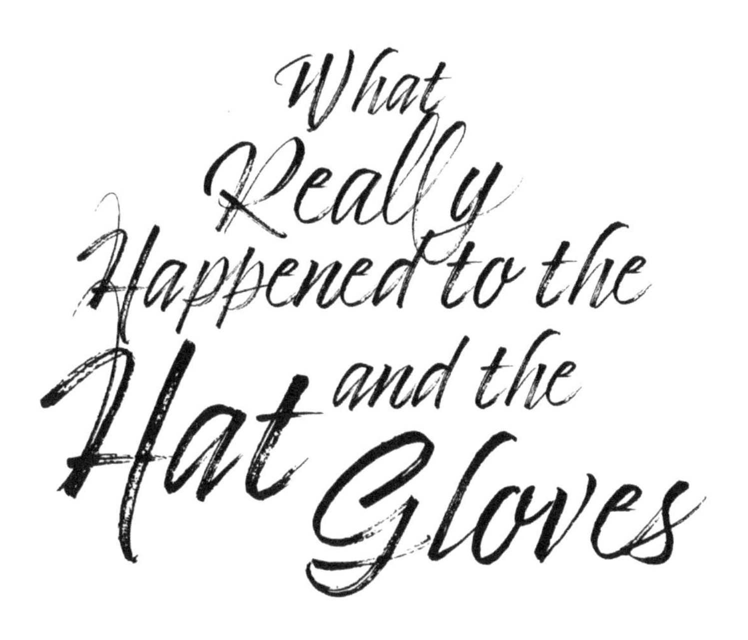

A True Story

CYNTHIA COOK

atmosphere press

Published by Atmosphere Press

Cover design by Felipe Betim

Atmospherepress.com

What really happened to the hat and the gloves?
It depends upon who you ask.

This is a true story.
The names and places have been changed.

Dedicated to my friend and family lawyer, Brenda Cameron,
for once again providing me with sound legal advice about
how to deal with my dysfunctional family.

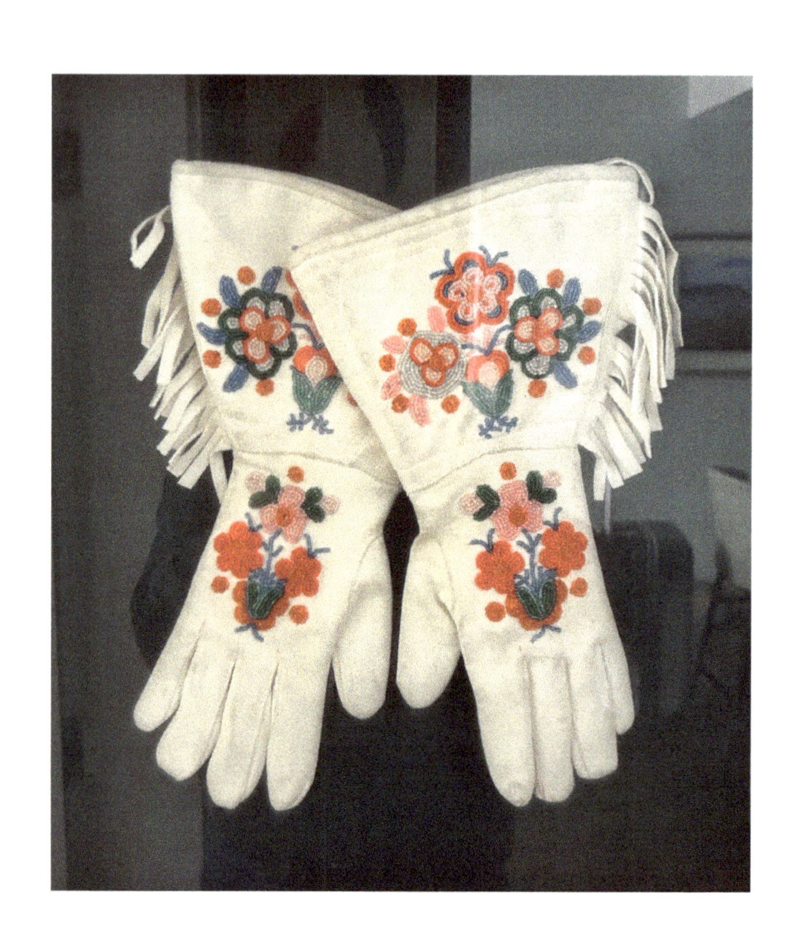

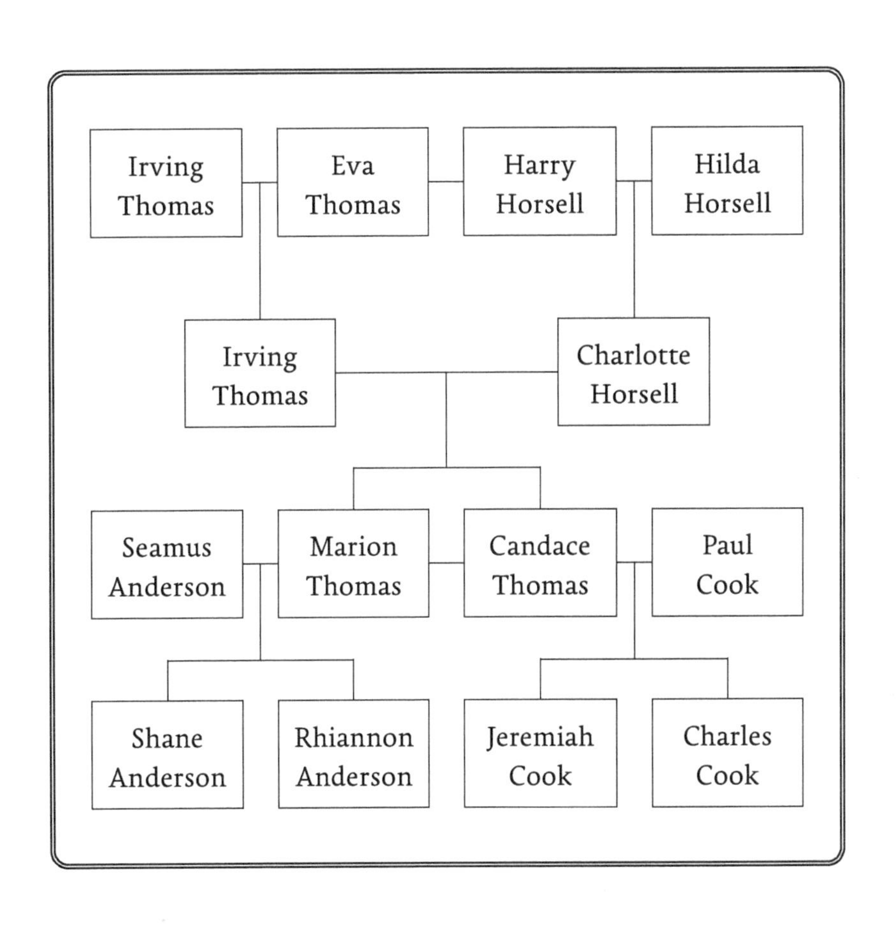
Irving Thomas
Eva Thomas
Harry Horsell
Hilda Horsell
Irving Thomas
Charlotte Horsell
Seamus Anderson
Marion Thomas
Candace Thomas
Paul Cook
Shane Anderson
Rhiannon Anderson
Jeremiah Cook
Charles Cook

Table of Contents

Chapter 1

Marion

I'm a wealthy single woman who has lived independently until recently. I have owned homes in Vancouver, Toronto, Gambier Island, Salt Spring Island, Squamish, Brackendale, and Park City on Vancouver Island. I have two adult children: a son, Shane, and a daughter, Rhiannon. I have no grandchildren. I was tall (five feet, eight inches) but now I'm only about five feet, four inches. My hair is grey and shoulder length. I have lost a lot of weight since I moved to Park City.

I recently moved in with my son, Shane, and his partner, Sunshine, to a new larger home in Park City. I am no longer able to live independently. My memory is impaired. I can't keep track of time. I'm constantly anxious about where my keys, credit cards, purse, and passport are. I don't know where my mother's diamond ring went. I never used to drink before, but the consumption of white wine has become my coping mechanism. I have mobility problems. I have poor vision due to cataracts, especially at night. I'm lonely, and sometimes I think that it would be better if I just died. I can't do most of the things I used to enjoy anymore, including quilting. My travel is limited. I trust almost nobody now.

I only have one sibling, Candace, who is five years younger than me. She is married to Paul, and they live in Burnaby. She has one surviving child, Charles, who resides in Vancouver. Candace has no grandchildren. My sister is still in good health and exhibits no sign of mental decline so far. Candace is the same age as our mother was when she died of a massive stroke.

Candace and her husband came to stay at my house in Park City, right before I moved in with my son and his partner. They were there under the guise of helping me and Shane, but Candace's real agenda was to take advantage of me in order to get a pair of gloves that were hand beaded by our maternal grandmother. Candace said she wanted them for Charles, but instead, my sister took them home to their apartment where she displayed them.

The most unforgivable act committed by Candace during her stay with me was the deliberate destruction of Sunshine's hat. It was done with willful and malicious intent to hurt Sunshine and Shane, and it did. My son had stopped by my house to discuss a few details pertaining to the move to our new shared home. Candace asked Shane about the hat and what the large plume of fur on it was. Shane told Candace, "It's Sunshine's hat, and the fur came from her deceased dog, who was irreplaceable to her." Candace told my son that she was glad she had asked him about the hat and to please return it to Sunshine, which he, unfortunately, didn't do. Later that night, I saw Candace beside my bankers desk near the hat with a pair of scissors in her hand. I can't remember why I didn't ask her what she was doing or why Paul didn't stop her.

Two days later, Shane returned to my house to take me to get a manicure and pedicure. My son discovered that the large plume of dog fur had been cut off to about two and a half inches and disposed of, although he didn't find it in the trash. Sunshine was devastated by her loss.

To make matters even worse, Candace and Paul have steadfastly continued to deny any knowledge of or wrongdoing to the hat, despite the obvious fact that they're the only ones who could have done it, because I'm an eyewitness. When Paul met with Shane (only Paul because my son won't see Candace) two months after the fact, Paul refused to admit that they were both lying.

Candace and Paul have continued to try to win back my affections by sending me a blanket featuring photographs of our children when they were younger, taken on a family vacation to Disneyland, and pictures of friends visiting the vacation home I owned on Gambier Island. Of course, I want nothing to do with either one of them after this betrayal. I refused to give Candace my new telephone number because she took the gloves under false pretenses. Candace hasn't even returned the photographs and memory book she borrowed from me as she promised. To think that Shane and I once said to Candace, "It would be so nice if Paul and you lived nearby in Park City!"

Sunshine doesn't want Candace to have our telephone number because of what she did to her hat. My son, Shane, has unfriended them both, and he has stopped replying to Paul's messages.

Chapter 2

Shane

I'm an honest, hardworking guy who lives in Park City with my partner, Sunshine, and my mom, Marion. Sunshine and I do everything we can to support my mom, who has Alzheimer's. It's a second full-time job for both of us.

I'm tall and good-looking, with a full head of wavy, brown, shoulder-length hair and a beard. I have experienced a bit of middle-aged spread though. I have no biological children. I have one married sister, Rhiannon, who helps out as much as she can, but she lives far away in the Cariboo region of British Columbia.

I was close to my uncle Paul. I looked up to him as a father figure until two months ago. Sunshine and I can't forgive my aunt Candace for what only she could have done to Sunshine's hat, and until Candace and Paul both admit that they lied about it, they are out of our lives.

Eight months ago, it became obvious to me that my mom could no longer live alone safely. She put her cell phone in the microwave. Her neighbours complained, of course. My mom's short-term memory is gone. She asked, "Where's Rhiannon?" when my sister was standing right in front of her. I don't know when she last had the prescription for her eye-wear updated. My mom's mobility is limited. She's only able to travel domestically and with our support. Most days she sits alone and drinks white wine while watching *The Crown* on repeat. My mom often says, "There must be a hole in this glass!" before she has finished drinking her wine. My mom is lonely, so Sunshine and I have adjusted our work schedules so that one of us is always home.

Two months ago, I foolishly invited my aunt and uncle to stay in Mom's old house to help her transition to our new shared living situation. At the time, it appeared that they had come with the best of intentions. Candace and Paul arrived bearing gifts of an orchid, wine, and beer. My mom had lost a lot of weight, so Candace helped her clean and organize her closet. My aunt worked in high-end retail, so she has a good eye for fashion. She helped my mom select new clothes in her size (ones that my mom can manage because she has trouble with buttons and zippers). Paul helped us move furniture in the new house. They both made sure that my mom had food in her fridge and either ordered take-out or took her out to eat. They even cut up her food for her, helped her to get dressed in the morning, and tucked her into bed at night. They ran several loads of my mom's laundry.

Candace did legitimately take the gloves, which had also been hand beaded by her Metis grandmother. My aunt said that they would pass to Charles eventually, not immediately. Candace received my mom's permission – and mine and Rhiannon's – to take the gloves. I don't know why it has become my mom's latest obsession. When Candace and Paul learned my mom had been saying that my aunt took advantage of her because Candace didn't immediately give the gloves to Charles but instead hung them up on their apartment wall, my aunt and uncle offered to return them. Then my mom did an about-face and said that Candace could keep the gloves for Charles.

As we speak, the hotly contested gloves are out of my aunt and uncle's storage locker and on their way back to their rightful owner, Charles. Now let's return to the important issue, the hat!

Late in the afternoon on the day before my aunt and uncle returned to Burnaby, I had stopped by my mom's house to take care of some business pertaining to her transition to our shared living situation. My aunt Candace asked me about Sunshine's hat and the large plume of dog hair. At the time, I thought it was because she was helping my mom declutter. I told Candace how important the hat, and especially the fur from Sunshine's deceased dog, was. Candace told me she was glad that she had asked me, and would I please take the hat back home to Sunshine. My only regret is that I didn't do as Candace wanted me to.

Two days later, I returned to my mom's house to take her to have a manicure and pedicure. That's when I discovered that the large plume of dog fur had been cut off with scissors to a length of about two and a half inches and disposed of. Unfortunately, I couldn't find the evidence.

Only six people had been in the house during the time my aunt and uncle stayed with my mom: Marion, me, Sunshine, Candace, Paul, and Sunshine's mother, Susie. To this day, none of them will admit to having committed this senseless act of destruction.

I don't usually go on Facebook, but I posted that someone had deliberately done something to hurt me, and it did. Uncle Paul was still one of my friends at the time, so he asked what my post was referring to. I told him that something had been done to Sunshine's hat. Paul said that he and Candace didn't know anything about it because neither one of them had ever touched the hat or looked at it again before they left my mom's house and went home.

I didn't communicate with my uncle again until a few weeks later when Paul messaged me to ask whether we had received the photo blanket they ordered from London Drugs and had shipped to us. I replied to my uncle that we had and I must not have hit send with the message I wrote to that effect. I wished Candace and Paul a happy Easter and said that it would have been even more special if they could have joined us for our first family dinner at our new house.

Everything changed a few weeks later when my mom said that she had seen my aunt Candace at her bankers desk near Sunshine's hat with a pair of scissors in her hand! I don't know why Paul didn't ask Candace what she was doing, or my mom didn't try to stop her sister. I'm surprised that Mom was able to clearly see what Candace was doing from ten feet away because her vision is poor, especially at night. But my mom's account of events must be accurate.

I immediately unfriended Candace on Facebook because she didn't deserve an opportunity to explain herself. In order to respect Sunshine's wishes, I didn't give our new telephone number to Candace when Paul asked for it.

When Paul and Candace returned home from their vacation, I messaged Paul to meet with him at the train station in Vancouver on the day I was travelling on the Rocky Mountaineer with Mom, Sunshine, and Rhiannon. I made it quite clear that Candace's presence was unwelcome. But my sister Rhiannon was in attendance.

I gave Paul every opportunity to admit that they were both lying because I know they were the only ones who could have taken the scissors to Sunshine's hat. I even tried emotional blackmail with the implied threat that if Paul and Candace didn't confess to what they must have done, the family picture would no longer include them. Paul continued to say that he and Candace will never confess to something they didn't do, so I have unfriended him and stopped replying to his messages.

This will be the first year that I won't telephone Uncle Paul on Father's Day because I no longer look up to him as a father figure.

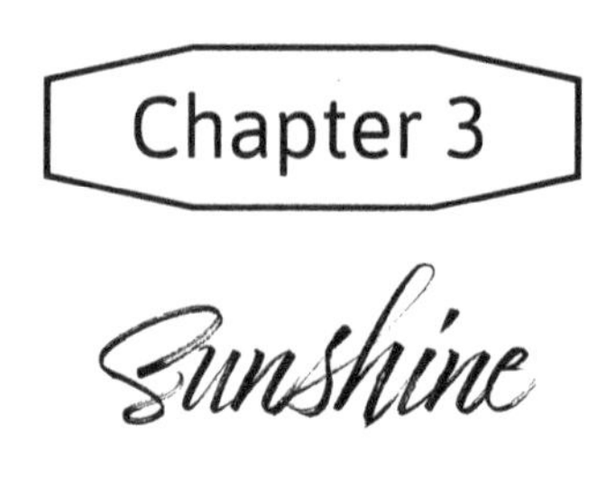

I work very hard as a geriatric care nurse, both at the hospital in Victoria and at home in Park City with Shane's mother, who has Alzheimer's. I have two adult children, Jack and Diane, from a previous relationship. Shane and I don't have any children together. I'm older than Shane. I have shoulder-length, brown hair, and I'm average height and weight. I wear my fingernails short because I take care of elderly patients who have fragile skin.

I'm the central character in this story because irreparable harm has been done to me by Shane's aunt Candace. I don't know why Candace would deliberately hurt me, because all I have done is love and support Shane and Marion. Until two months ago, I thought that all Candace wanted to do was help all three of us but I was wrong.

I wasn't a witness to any of these events but I support Shane in believing his mother's eyewitness account of his aunt taking scissors to my hat. I'll never know why Candace did it and then left the evidence of the hat on Marion's bankers desk, or where my dog's fur went.

Shane, Marion, and I never want them to communicate with us through any means.

Chapter 4

Rhiannon

I'm married to the love of my life. Finn is younger than me. He's tall, handsome, and incredibly kind. Family is everything to him. I'm the luckiest girl in the world! Finn and I live in the Cariboo. Neither of us has ever had children. It's not easy for me to travel anywhere except Edmonton, so I don't get to see my mother as often as I would like to or to be there to support my brother, Shane, and his partner, Sunshine, as much as I should.

I really wish that Shane hadn't involved me in his drama. I messaged my cousin Charles to say that I disagreed with her cousin Shane about the rightful ownership of the hand-beaded gloves. I still want Candace and my uncle Paul to stay in my life, and it was very unpleasant to hear my brother make accusations and implied threats to my uncle in my aunt's absence. Shane didn't get the confession he was after, even when he kept repeating that Candace and Paul were both lying because he knew they were guilty, and they had to admit it. Shane never said how he knew that Candace and Paul were the only ones who could have taken the scissors to Sunshine's hat, what he thought their motive was, when they had the opportunity to do this heinous act, or where the evidence of the dog fur was. Interestingly, Uncle Paul's version of events corroborates Aunt Candace's account of the hat incident, that neither of them knew anything about it.

The end result is the same, though. I am going to see my aunt and uncle far less often because they will be excluded from family celebrations. I'm glad that Finn and I were married two years ago, so that we have pictures to prove we all had fun together.

I will always miss my cousin Jeremiah, who had to leave us nine years ago. I haven't seen my cousin Charles since Jeremiah's celebration of life. I hadn't even met Finn at the time. Finn still hasn't met Charles, who couldn't attend our wedding due to work obligations.

I've been happily married to my awesome wife, Rhiannon, for two years, but we met five years ago. My wife is fearless and beautiful in an unconventional way. She often wears streaks in her hair in her favorite colour, purple. Rhiannon has several tattoos, which all have special meanings.

I have lived in the Cariboo my whole life. My mother was widowed young, so I have supported her as much as possible.

Rhiannon has a great attitude and sense of humour. We have lots of fun living with many rescued dogs and a cat.

I have gotten to know my aunt and uncle since we all partied together at my wedding. Candace told me how much their son, Jeremiah, would have loved to be there. I replied, "Thank you for accepting me."

I hope that I get to meet Charles someday because we're about the same age.

Chapter 6

Charles

I live and work in Vancouver, where I'm assistant program director at a museum. My degree is in original works, so I still perform in, write for, and direct theatre part-time. I'm happy in a long-distance relationship. I have no children. I'm the only surviving child of Paul and Candace. We lost my brother, Jeremiah, nine years ago, the same month I graduated from university. He never had the chance to have children, so Paul and Candace have no grandchildren.

I'm an unconventional person. I have short, chestnut-coloured hair. I'm five feet, six inches tall, with a slim athletic build because I ride my bike everywhere. I look like my mother did when she was young. My parents have always supported me in everything I've done and have been proud of my accomplishments. The first thing they did when Candace got her inheritance was to repay my student loans. My brother and I attended private school in Vancouver, even though it meant that my parents both had to make personal sacrifices.

My happiest childhood memories are of the times my brother and I spent with my parents, my aunt Marion, and my cousins, Shane and Rhiannon. Jeremiah loved his aunt Marion and his cousins very much. There are portraits of us together taken at my aunt's Salt Spring home. We have informal pictures of us which were taken at our summer cabins on

Gambier Island and on joint family vacations in Disneyland during happier times.

I had dinner with my parents last night at their apartment. I'm now in possession of my great-grandmother's hand-beaded gloves, which I recognize as original Cree artwork. My parents had taken them off their apartment wall when allegations were made by my aunt that my mother had acquired them fraudulently.

I have never known either of my parents to lie about anything. In fact, my mother is brutally honest. I have never witnessed my mother senselessly destroy anyone's property or take anything without permission.

I guess I won't be seeing my cousin Shane anymore. I'm sorry that I didn't see my aunt Marion more often while she was still lucid, but at least I got to say goodbye last Christmas.

I hope that I can stay in my cousin Rhiannon's life and that someday I will meet her husband, Finn.

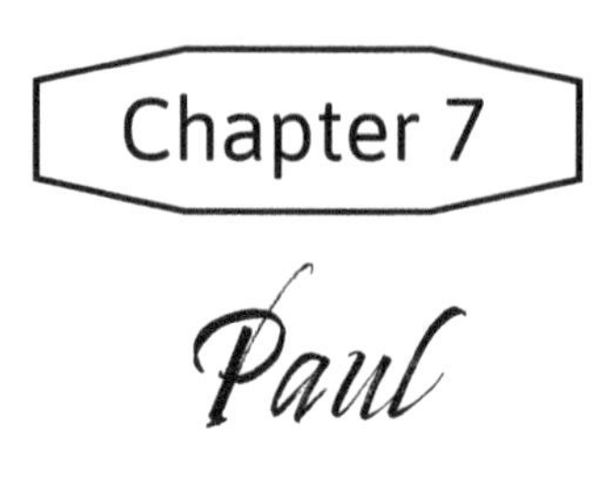

Chapter 7

Paul

I'm a retired, usually very patient man. I'm tall and in good physical health because my wife makes us live a healthy lifestyle, including regular exercise! I've been married to Candace for forty-five years, so I think that I know her better than anyone else does. We live in Burnaby near our only surviving child. The loss of our son, Jeremiah, nine years ago is a wound that time hasn't healed. We have no grandchildren.

Candace and I both got new prescription eyewear early this year so that we can see clearly. Neither of us has any symptoms of Alzheimer's yet. Candace and I enjoy travelling and going to rock concerts. We are active, watch our diets, and usually avoid alcohol. We go to fitness classes regularly, paddleboard, hike, and snorkel. We never miss our doctor or dentist appointments.

We first noticed my sister-in-law, Marion, behaving strangely nine years ago while we still lived in Squamish and she resided in Brackendale with her daughter, Rhiannon, and her then-husband, Ty. Soon after Jeremiah's death, Rhiannon and Ty separated. Rhiannon was in a relationship with a man my sister-in-law disapproved of, so Marion abruptly kicked Rhiannon out of their house and stopped speaking to her. That's when Rhiannon moved up to the Cariboo where she met her husband, Finn, a few years later.

The only thing Marion seemed to miss was Rhiannon's

Buddha head, which had been hanging on my sister-in-law's wall. At the time, Marion told Candace that she had disinherited Rhiannon, which wasn't well received by my wife. My sister-in-law also announced her intention to spend all her money on the Brackendale property so that there would be no liquid assets remaining in her estate for Shane and Rhiannon to contest. Marion had also purchased a Raku figurine of two birds from the thrift shop and said that it represented her two children fighting over a worm. Marion stated that Shane and Rhiannon wished that she was already dead so they could have the proceeds of her estate immediately.

Candace and I met Sunshine once in 2015 before Shane and his new partner moved to Park City. We didn't see Sunshine again for seven years, until Rhiannon and Finn's wedding.

Twenty fifteen was also the year Charles graduated from university in Seattle. Charles made both of us proud by achieving cum laude honours. We naturally told Charles's aunt. Charles lived in Seattle for another year under the university's Optional Training Program, which allowed non-US citizens to work in their area of study, which was theatre and performance.

Twenty fifteen was when my father-in-law, Irving, passed away, one week after Jeremiah's death. Irving never honoured his promise to help Jeremiah, although with my father-in-law's wealth he could have done so anytime he wanted to. When Irving was on his deathbed, Marion told Candace not to visit him because Irving didn't want to see my wife. Shane visited his grandfather regularly, and Rhiannon went to see him with Marion too. After Irving's death, my sister-in-law told Candace that she wouldn't inherit because his whole estate had been spent on his care.

We couldn't learn the terms of Irving's will right away because it was hidden in a trust. Our family lawyer and friend told us that he'd done it to screw Candace. My wife replied that it wouldn't be the first time but to tell his new family that Candace was prepared to fight until all the money was gone. Suddenly, my wife learned that she and my sister-in-law would inherit. The first disbursement was made that year. Candace immediately repaid Charles's student loans.

In 2016, my sister-in-law took advantage of Candace and me to sell her recreational property on Gambier Island. We provided all of the transportation to and from our vacation homes. We did all the maintenance and heavy lifting around her cabin, in addition to our own. Marion even rode to and from the dock to her home on the gator, while Candace walked. She never kept a barbecue there, so dinner, and usually lunch, was always at our cabin.

We had been trying to sell our cabin since Jeremiah died because there were too many memories of both our children growing up. Our property was reasonably priced, but my sister-in-law came in at a much lower price because she had stopped paying her strata fees over a dispute with her co-owners. Lucy Bowman grew up enjoying summers on Gambier Island on her parents' recreational property. Lucy had returned with her husband and three young children because she wanted to purchase another island home for them.

Lucy stopped by our place one day while my sister-in-law was over, as she usually was. Lucy said she wanted to view our cabin and that she would inform us of her decision either way. Then she went back to Marion's place to have a look.

It became clear to us that Lucy had made an offer on my sister-in-law's property. Valuable items started disappearing from her cabin, such as heavy, teak deck chairs that we hadn't helped her take back home. Suddenly, a barbecue appeared in her shed. Lucy never even telephoned our Realtor to tell us that she had decided against purchasing our cabin.

Marion went on a cruise to Alaska that fall with her then-closest friend, Sherry, from Salt Spring Island. My sister-in-law has since stopped speaking to Sherry too. Candace and I had been invited for drinks at one of Marion's neighbour's home. In front of almost all the strata owners, one of our close neighbour's adult son announced that Lucy had purchased Marion's cabin despite all the unpaid strata fees. Another of Marion's neighbours much more politely said that Lucy had announced it on the water taxi over to Gambier Island. The next morning, we removed our kayaks from Marion's shed before Lucy took possession of her new property.

Lucy got a real bargain on Marion's cabin, which was priced at only $280,000. My sister-in-law's stated objective had been to drive down every other property owner's resale price on their cabins. We would have put some of the money we inherited from Irving towards purchasing our co-owners' bare lot and paying off the unpaid strata fees that had accrued for a year. Marion probably would have seen $500,000 from the real estate transaction, and we would have congratulated her instead of feeling betrayed. Strata Council members were mad at her too over the unpaid fees. The next two summers were some of our most enjoyable ones because we only had one property to maintain!

Fast forward to 2017, our last Christmas in Squamish, and our first Christmas without either of our children. Marion told us that she preferred Christmas without Shane and Rhiannon. Candace and I celebrated the next four Christmases with just the two of us.

In 2018, we sold our property in Squamish and purchased an apartment in Burnaby. We also sold our cabin on Gambier Island and saw more money for it than Marion did in 2016. We stopped seeing Marion in 2018 and sought counseling, on Charles's advice, to deal with our childhood trauma. Candace got her money's worth on the second session when the therapist said, "Your sister obviously always has to be right. You can be right or you can be in a relationship."

Fast forward to 2022, the next time we saw Marion. The family had gathered to celebrate the joyous occasion of Rhiannon and Finn's wedding. Candace and I were both shocked to see how much Marion had aged. She managed the stairs with difficulty. We both made the mistake of feeling sorry for Marion and let her back into our lives. We didn't know that she was still quite capable of doing terrible things to us. This time the harm she caused to our relationship with our nephew, Shane, was irreparable and unforgivable. I wish we could have seen what was coming a year and a half later.

Beginning in 2022, we maintained contact with Marion by telephone. Things were quite pleasant, although we began to notice that my sister-in-law didn't seem to be as mentally sharp. We visited Marion's Park City home for the first time in 2023. Marion's home was beautiful, and we enjoyed seeing Shane and Sunshine too. But we definitely began to notice that Marion was in a bit of a fog at times. We were both shocked to see her drinking because she had never done that before. The next time we saw Charles, Candace said, "If you want to see your aunt again, you had better come to Park City with us." Charles told us that they would join us on our next visit because Charles did want to see Marion again.

Candace and I were invited for Thanksgiving by our nephew, Shane. We were both concerned by how much weight Marion had lost. Candace has a family history of Alzheimer's, so there was no mistaking the symptoms. Our nephew told us that Marion's rapid mental decline had started the previous month, which was when my sister-in-law put her cell phone in the microwave. Shane had signing authorization on Marion's bank account because my sister-in-law could no longer manage her finances. That's when Marion asked Candace and me to take over the task of liquidating the family business because she couldn't stay on top of it anymore.

Candace and I returned to Park City two months later with Charles. Marion hadn't seen Charles for seven years, so we hoped my sister-in-law appreciated the visit.

Candace and I went to Park City again in early 2024 when Rhiannon and Finn were able to visit. We had a fun family vacation with them, Marion, Shane, and Sunshine, but it was definitely tinged with sadness too.

Our nephew, Shane, asked us to stay with Marion two months later, to help her transition to their new joint living arrangement. Candace would keep Marion company and help her to clean and organize her closet and select new clothes in the right size for my sister-in-law. Candace attempted to clear clutter in a sincere effort to help with their move. I helped Shane and Sunshine move furniture into their new house. It was beautiful, and it was such a relief to us to know that Marion wouldn't be alone so much. Shane said he and Sunshine never thought that they would own anything like their new home. Candace congratulated her nephew on how well they had done. We both imagined all three of them living with much less stress. Shane offered us a place to stay anytime. I guess that offer has expired.

In hindsight, we never should have taken the gloves. Marion, Shane, and Rhiannon had all said that Candace could have them. Once again, my wife thought she was helping because they wouldn't have to move the gloves to the new house. Now we see the error of our ways. We should have known how agitated Marion would become when she realized that the gloves were missing because we had taken them home with us. Paranoia is a common symptom of Alzheimer's, the perception that people have come to visit them with the sole purpose of stealing their valuables.

I never heard Candace tell Marion that the gloves would pass immediately to Charles, but my sister-in-law became obsessed with the idea that Candace had taken advantage of her when Marion saw that we had displayed the gloves on our Burnaby apartment wall. Two months later, Shane told us what Marion had been saying about Candace to explain why his mother didn't want my wife to have their telephone number. Candace immediately offered to return the gloves to Marion. After we had already taken the gloves down and put them in our storage locker, Marion said that Candace could keep them for Charles.

The story of the hotly contested ownership of the hand-beaded gloves has concluded with us giving them to Charles at our first opportunity. Even this will probably never satisfy Marion.

Now to the sordid story of Sunshine's hat. What really happened to the hat? Candace and I honestly don't know what, if anything, happened to Sunshine's hat and the large plume of fur from Sunshine's deceased dog. How we inadvertently involved ourselves in this mess was a sincere effort to help Marion declutter. Candace really regrets ever having seen the hat sitting on Marion's bankers desk and asking Shane about it. Shane told Candace that the hat was Sunshine's prized possession and that the tiny tuft of fluff that we both saw, wearing our new prescription eyeglasses, had belonged to Sunshine's deceased dog, which was irreplaceable to her. Candace told her nephew she was glad that she had asked him about it, and would he please return the hat to Sunshine. Unfortunately, he didn't, and Shane must not have even looked at it because neither Candace nor I ever saw a large plume of dog fur on it or found it in the kitchen trash.

Before Candace and I returned to Burnaby the next morning, we took Marion out for breakfast. True to her word, my wife never touched, or even looked at, Sunshine's hat again. Sunshine was a witness to none of these events.

Late in the afternoon two days later, Shane returned to his mother's house to take her to have a manicure and pedicure. That's when Shane told me that something had been done to Sunshine's hat. I told my nephew that we honestly didn't know anything about it.

Before Candace and I left on our vacation, we ordered a blanket from London Drugs, using her cherished photos, and had it delivered to their new Park City home. We telephoned Marion to say goodbye and to wish them all good luck with their move. My sister-in-law was happy to hear from us, and we thought that we were all on good terms.

About two weeks later, I messaged Shane to ask him whether they had received the blanket. I got a delivery notice, but I was surprised that our nephew hadn't mentioned the blanket. Shane replied that they had received the blanket; he thought he had messaged me, but he must have forgotten to hit send. He said that Marion had moved into their new home and was having difficulty with the transition, which was to be expected. My nephew told me what he had planned for their first family dinner in their new shared home, and that he wished Candace and I could attend.

Candace and I continued to purchase gifts for Marion, Shane, and Sunshine during our travels, which we thought would be appreciated. A few weeks later, I received a cryptic message from Shane. He said that his mom was upset. I replied that Marion must have had difficulty adjusting to the move from her old house. Shane replied that wasn't what Marion was upset about, but he didn't elaborate.

When Candace and I returned to Burnaby after our vacation, we asked Shane for their new telephone number so that Candace could call her sister to wish Marion happy travels on the Rocky Mountaineer with her children and Sunshine. My nephew replied that he would meet with me, but not with his aunt, for coffee at the train station.

Candace asked me not to discuss anything pertaining to her sister in my wife's absence. I waited for Shane at the train station for ten minutes before he made an appearance with our niece, Rhiannon, in tow! Rhiannon sat silently during our conversation, but she was obviously very uncomfortable and didn't agree with anything my nephew said. At least she is a reliable witness who can corroborate my account of this event.

Shane began by explaining why Marion didn't want Candace to have their telephone number. My sister-in-law had become fixated on the idea that Candace had taken the hand-beaded gloves under false pretenses. Marion claimed that my wife had told my sister-in-law that the gloves would be given directly to Charles. I was present during the whole time the ownership of the gloves was discussed and remember no such conversation. My sister-in-law became upset when she saw a picture of the gloves hanging on our apartment wall. Marion said that Candace had taken advantage of her to obtain possession of the gloves, which had also belonged to my wife's grandmother, Hilda.

Then Shane continued by explaining why Sunshine didn't want his aunt to have their new phone number. Apparently, it had been decided that Candace and I were the only ones who could have cut the large plume of dog fur off Sunshine's hat and disposed of it (although for some reason, not in Marion's kitchen trash can). Sunshine was not a witness to any of these events. Candace and I are the only credible witnesses to these events, both being of sound mind and both wearing our new prescription eyewear.

I obviously strenuously refuted all of these accusations. I pointed out that it wasn't right that Candace wasn't present to defend herself. I told Shane that we had no motive to commit this senseless act of property damage because we only know Sunshine as my sister-in-law's primary caregiver. I pointed out that we had no opportunity to do what we had been accused of and that we never touched or even looked at Sunshine's hat after my nephew instructed Candace not to. I also mentioned that neither one of us, with our good vision, had ever even seen a large plume of dog fur on Sunshine's hat, only a tuft about two and a half inches long, which had not been evenly cut by scissors.

It was an exercise in futility to tell my nephew anything. He continued to insist that Candace and I were both lying. We knew it, and we had to admit it, because we were the only ones who could have taken scissors to Sunshine's hat. The unspoken threat was that neither one of us would be part of their family unless we confessed.

nded abruptly when I told my nephew
imstances would his aunt and uncle ever
ing we hadn't done. Shane has no physical
port his accusations, and we are two compe-
who deny wrongdoing. I told my nephew that
uld be livid, and she was.

ane had already unfriended Candace on Facebook, but the next time my nephew messaged me was when he saw my post, which read, "Mistreating people and then avoiding communication with them isn't 'protecting your peace,' it's avoiding accountability." He also read Candace's comment, "Not what you would expect from a 44-year-old man." My nephew messaged me to apologize for causing pain by repeating what his mom had said, but that we shouldn't shoot the messenger.

I replied to my nephew, stating what terms and conditions his aunt and uncle would apply to a relationship with Shane and Sunshine moving forward. Shane and Sunshine both had to stop saying things about Candace and me that weren't true unless he could provide evidence to support his accusations. We both knew that he couldn't because it never happened, and even if it did, the deed was done before Candace and I ever saw Sunshine's precious hat.

I told Shane that he and Sunshine had every right to refuse to see Candace, but they had absolutely no right to prevent his aunt from seeing her sister.

Shane replied, "OK, that's fair enough, I have no proof, but how would you explain what happened to Sunshine's hat when I didn't do it, Sunshine didn't do it, Susie didn't do it, and my mom didn't do it?" Obviously, my nephew is no legal expert. The burden of proof is on the accuser, not the defendant, who is presumed innocent until proven guilty. The credible witnesses, Candace and I, have corroborated each other's recollection of events, that neither one of us ever touched the hat again after Shane told Candace not to.

My sister-in-law lacks the capacity to be a credible witness, due to her Alzheimer's, alcoholism, and poor vision,

especially at night. But Shane messaged me that Ma[illegible]
him that she had seen Candace near Sunshine's hat wi[illegible]
pair of scissors in her hand. I wish that I had believed my wife when she told me that it must have been Marion who said that Candace cut the dog fur off Sunshine's hat. My sister-in-law didn't explain why she didn't try to stop Candace from taking scissors to Sunshine's hat.

Shane said that he would have Marion call her sister when they returned home. I told my nephew that Candace didn't want Marion to call, and so far, she hasn't.

I messaged my nephew that neither my wife nor I ever wanted to hear another word about Sunshine's hat. I said to Shane, "There's no fricking way that Candace and I will ever confess to something we didn't do." That's when my nephew unfriended me too and stopped replying to my messages.

I guess I won't be getting my annual telephone call from Shane this Father's Day. It's no great loss. I never raised any children who would have called their aunt and uncle liars and told them that they had to admit it, in their aunt's absence but in front of their niece.

Why was Sunshine so quick to accept Marion's account of what happened to the hat? Because Sunshine doesn't know our family either. Sunshine had never even met Charles when she asked whether Charles's degree was ever completed. The only person who could have told Sunshine that was my sister-in-law. It's hardly the action of an aunt taking pride in Charles's accomplishment of graduating cum laude nine years ago.

Candace and I are no longer sympathetic towards Marion, and neither one of us wants to help my sister-in-law anymore. My wife and I aren't considering relocating to Park City in the future.

Candace has now done everything she said that she would do and nothing that she said she wouldn't. Charles returned home with the gloves after the first time Charles visited our apartment. We received a notice of delivery of Marion's photographs and memory book to their new address, plus a choice letter to Shane that he doubtless hasn't had the courage to open. That's fine, because I made a copy of it for Charles. We notified Rhiannon that the memory book was returned to her mother.

Shane eventually replied to my message, acknowledging receipt of the package. My nephew said he hadn't responded because he didn't think anyone in my household wanted to hear from him. Shane was right about that. Candace and I only wanted to make sure that Rhiannon would receive her mother's Christmas memory book as his sister had said she wanted it. There were obviously no thank-yous or recognition of the fact that the photographs and memory book were returned to Marion as promised by Candace. There was no acknowledgement of the photograph I sent Shane of Charles displaying the gloves in Charles's apartment, in accordance with his mother's wishes. In Shane's unique personal style, he saw this message as an opportunity to tell me how hard his life was with his two jobs (caring for his mother and the work that he is paid for). Nobody had asked how any of them were, and Shane never inquired about how any of the people in my household were.

Chapter 8

Candace

I'm an active senior. I will be fully retired next year after I have completed the task of liquidating the family business. I live in Burnaby with Paul, my husband of forty-five years. We have one surviving adult child, Charles, who lives and works in Vancouver. Our son, Jeremiah, passed away nine years ago. We have no grandchildren.

Paul and I work out almost every day. I'm petite and slim, with long, straight, blonde hair. I have several tattoos, all of which have meaning. We hike, paddleboard, and snorkel. We enjoy travelling and attending rock concerts.

I got new prescription eyewear in January, and I take AREDS to preserve my vision. So far, I exhibit no symptoms of Alzheimer's. I'm careful about my diet and avoid alcohol because of my family history of stroke and Alzheimer's disease. I have a brain scan done every five years.

Anyone who knows me well would tell you that I'm nobody's fool and disarmingly honest. I don't do senseless, self-destructive acts of damage to other people's property. I would never take advantage of a senior or someone with a hidden disability, such as autism, for my own personal gain. Inclusion is the cause I fundraise for, in memory of Jeremiah.

I can corroborate Paul's account of all the events I was present for as a credible witness. I was excluded from the meeting at the train station where my nephew called us both liars and said that we had to admit it. Fortunately, Paul didn't confess to something we hadn't done, and our niece was present as a credible witness.

My nephew's accusations are baseless. He has no credible witness or physical evidence to support his account of what really happened to the hat. There's no motive and no opportunity. The two credible witnesses never saw a large plume of dog fur on Sunshine's hat or saw any dog fur in Marion's kitchen trash.

I'm not calling my sister a liar because she has Alzheimer's. Hallucinations are a part of dementia. Events can be combined to create an alternative memory. My sister could have seen me in the kitchen, using scissors to cut the tags off her new clothes. On a separate occasion, I was at her bankers desk near Sunshine's hat, but without scissors in my hand.

I can't forgive my sister for this betrayal because it is the worst thing she's ever done to me. My relationship with my nephew is broken beyond repair.

I only know Sunshine as my sister's primary caregiver, so what would motivate me to do Sunshine harm? If I had done this senseless act, why would I leave the evidence lying around? If Paul had seen me with a pair of scissors in my hand near Sunshine's hat, he would have prevented me from cutting the dog fur off it.

Why would I do this malicious act and then keep purchasing and sending gifts to these people? This is the craziest story that's been invented about me in fifty years.

Here is what I have learned from my nephew, Shane, and relearned from my sister, Marion, during the last two weeks:

1. No good deed goes unpunished.
2. When I have decided that someone is out of my life, under no circumstances should they be allowed back in.

3. You can remove someone's name from your will in one phone call to your lawyer.
4. No matter what you do for people who are truly ungrateful, they will never be satisfied.
5. Sometimes your worst enemy has been sitting beside you the whole time, disguised as a trusted family member.
6. Believe half of what you see and none of what you hear.
7. People don't change, they only get more so.
8. History repeats itself.
9. I don't have to love people just because they're family.
10. Everybody is a villain in someone's story.
11. You can't take it with you. If anyone could, my father would have done it.
12. Even Ted Bundy was allowed to present his own defense before he was sentenced to the death penalty.

The only thing I can agree on with my nephew is that I shouldn't see my sister because my presence only seems to further agitate Marion in her already confused mental state. I won't visit her at their home because of my instinct for self-preservation. Next time I might be accused of a serious crime like stealing her jewelry, such as our mother's diamond ring. She obviously doesn't remember giving it to Rhiannon, whom we saw wearing it at her wedding to Finn.

There are a lot of people in this world who are totally fine with causing unnecessary collateral damage as long as it helps them reach their goals. I'm just not one of them.

I can't believe what my nephew has become: ignorant, dishonest, disrespectful, selfish, and ungrateful. His communication skills could stand some improvement too. I don't love him anymore. If I ever see Shane again, it will only be in passing, and I won't speak to him. Next month, I'll start deleting any memories that mention Shane, Sunshine, or my sister.

I grew up in a house with my parents, my only sibling, Marion, and my widowed grandmother, Hilda (the one who hand beaded the gloves). My grandmother must have had early onset Alzheimer's because her memory was impaired, and she did many repetitive behaviors such as constantly looking for her purse and checking the contents. My grandmother lived to be ninety-four years old, but she hadn't recognized any of us as ourselves in at least twenty-five years. If I looked familiar, she would mistake me for a distant relative from thirty years ago. Towards the end of my mother's life, my grandmother thought that her daughter was a sister.

The only person my grandmother never forgot was her sister, Helena. That's why I think someday Marion might ask for me. I'll come to see her if anyone bothers to notify me.

If I learn that Marion is on her deathbed, I'll come to say goodbye. I'd like to see Shane and Sunshine try to stop me. The same thing goes if I learn that there will be a celebration of my sister's life. I'll put in an appearance, have one glass of wine, greet Rhiannon and Finn, and leave without speaking to Shane or Sunshine.

I can't imagine a worse fate than being remembered the way my sister has become. I want nothing that reminds me of her memory.

What really happened to the hat and the gloves?

I'll let the reader reach their own conclusions.

There are several sides to every story, depending upon how many people are involved either directly or indirectly. There are nine sides to this story: the truth, Marion's, Shane's, Sunshine's, Rhiannon's, Finn's, Charles's, Paul's, and mine.

I have written my story because the treatment that Paul and I have received from Marion and Shane is undeserved. If anything had happened to my sister, Paul and I would have taken Rhiannon and Shane in without hesitation. We would have found a way to make it work and raise them with Charles and Jeremiah.

Paul and I have been nothing but kind and generous to Marion and Shane (his whole life)! I know that my sister isn't in control of her actions anymore, but it's not exactly the first time that I've been made the family scapegoat. Shane and his partner, Sunshine (the geriatric care nurse), have obviously used undue influence to get Marion to say these terrible lies about me. As a consequence, my sister has lost my support and companionship, which she badly needs. I'm actually the only family member who stands to gain nothing from Marion.

Eventually, Shane will realize how much he's lost without his aunt, uncle, and cousin in his life. But Sunshine knows exactly what she's done to all of us. She hasn't so much as confronted me with her accusations as the owner of the hat should have. Sunshine wasn't even a witness to any of these events.

Perfect karma for all three of them is that they live together. Every day is Alzheimer's Groundhog Day with no more respite care from Paul and me.

The End

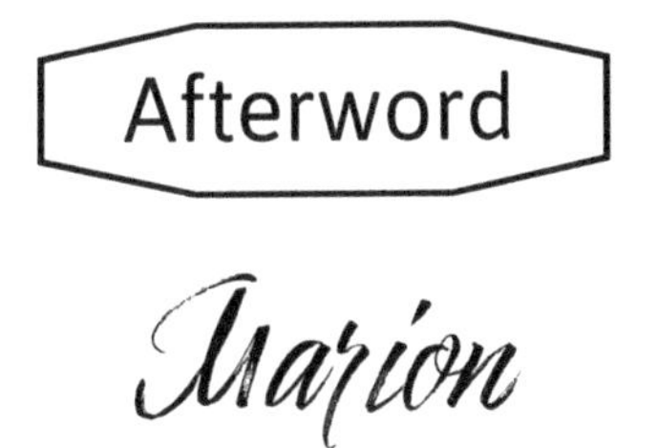

Afterword

Marion

(January 5, 1952-)

I'm at peace now, freed from the confusion and anxiety caused by Alzheimer's. I'll be remembered, and my story will be told by my children, Shane and Rhiannon.

I can't understand why my sister Candace never came to say goodbye to me. I've missed her so much. Maybe we will meet again in our next lives.

Resources

If you or someone you know needs support,
contact The Alzheimer's Society of BC
at 1-800-667-3742, or info@alzheimerbc.org

About Atmosphere Press

Founded in 2015, Atmosphere Press was built on the principles of Honesty, Transparency, Professionalism, Kindness, and Making Your Book Awesome. As an ethical and author-friendly hybrid press, we stay true to that founding mission today.

If you're a reader, enter our giveaway for a free book here:

SCAN TO ENTER
BOOK GIVEAWAY

If you're a writer, submit your manuscript for consideration here:

SCAN TO SUBMIT
MANUSCRIPT

And always feel free to visit Atmosphere Press and our authors online at atmospherepress.com. See you there soon!

About the Author

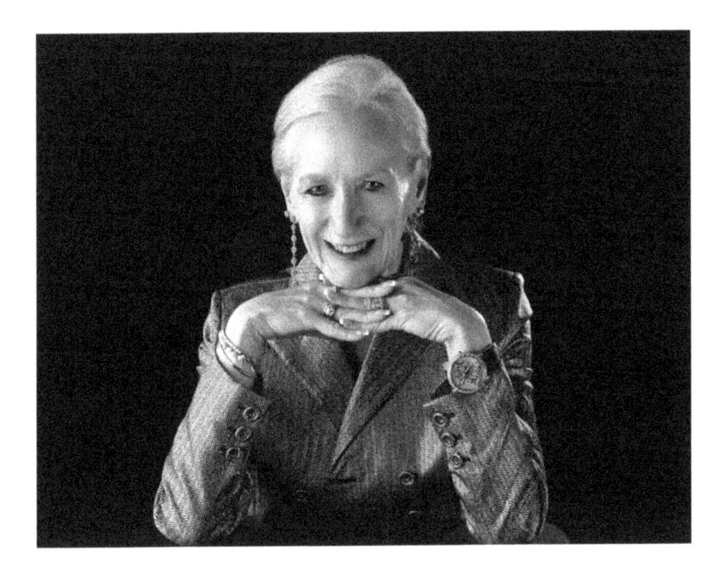

Cynthia Cook's first written work was in market research, in engineering and sales. She has written many papers on subjects including Taxonomy, Entomology, Plant Diseases, and Landscaping as an Advanced Master Gardener at VanDusen, Vancouver. This is Cynthia's first nonfiction novella. She has written from personal experience about the impact Alzheimer's can have on the person affected, their closest relatives, and caregivers.

www.ingramcontent.com/pod-product-compliance
Ingram Content Group UK Ltd.
Pitfield, Milton Keynes, MK11 3LW, UK
UKHW020820171224
452405UK00019B/138